Compilation of Herbs and Supplements for the Symptoms of Tick-Borne Diseases

By

Judy Wolf Lazzara

Compilation of Herbs and Supplements for the Symptoms of Tick-Borne Diseases

Judy Wolf Lazzara

TABLE OF CONTENT

DEDICATION

This book is dedicated to all those suffering, some for many years, with diseases that are not understood or dealt with by the mainstream medical community.

FOREWARD AND DISCLAIMER

First of all, this is not a medical report as I am not an acting medical professional. Check with your medical professional/provider with anything mentioned in this book.

I have used at one time or another, depending on symptoms, 99% of the supplements in this report. I am not "cured", or even in remission, but am able to lead as normal a life as possible with the help of the herbs and supplements. As many with Lyme and coinfections know, each day can be different with changing symptoms. There are some supplements/herbs I use on a daily basis, and others I rotate depending on need. I definitely try to protect the organs that can be negatively affected by the diseases.

I went through 6 months plus of antibiotics with the original infection, and more with later infections, that include Lyme, Anaplasma, Erlichia, Bartonella and Mycoplasma. Those antibiotics really messed up my digestive system. A few things with antibiotics got better, but many didn't. Since my background is in natural health, I felt I had to find a more favorable direction for my body. I was originally diagnosed with Lyme 10 years ago, but feel I have had it for over 20 years. After more than 20+ years of natural health schooling, DNA classes and extensive research, I have quite a list of supplements/herbs that have helped me. Stephen Harrod Buhner, William Rawls, Bryan Rosner, William Cowden, Richard Horowitz, teachers, and many others have helped to point me in the right directions, and I will be forever grateful for their contributions to the Lyme Community.

Originally, I decided to put this information down in a report form for myself to make dealing with symptom decisions easier. Then I had the thought that many other people looking for answers might find the information useful in their search of what works for them. As we all know, one size never fits all when it comes to dealing with these infections. I polled a couple of the groups I belong to and found interest in getting my research to the public. This can act as a head start for someone recently diagnosed; many trying to use a more natural way; and an adjunct to those on antibiotics who have been looking for answers for specific symptoms. I advise everyone to use this information to help guide their own research.

Most herbs have an overlap of what they can do for the body. Herbs contain so many different chemical compounds that more than one symptom may be covered. My suggestion would be to write down all, or your main, symptoms and see what particular herb(s) would cover or match the most symptoms at that time. I do that and it makes my decision easier.

As with most things, while a supplement might be a lifesaver for one person, it may not help another or even cause a problem for yet others. For that reason, I will usually start with a couple drops of a tincture, cut a pill in half or quarters, and even dump out half of a capsule, depending on the recommended dosage. Most tick-borne diseases can cause Herxheimer reactions from killing the bugs, so this is another reason to go slow and build up to recommended dosages.

As well as the supplements, I use a PEMF machine, Fremedica Wave-1 device and a portable sauna, that I feel have been useful. Not endorsements, but have seemed to help me!

Until the mainstream medical establishment can take our condition seriously, we are on our own looking for answers, sharing what has helped and giving as much support as we can to one another. LLMD's are hard to find, hard to get into and very expensive. I'm hoping that with so much long-haul Covid being in the news, doctors won't turn their back on that also, and find some answers for all of us. They found a "cocktail" for AIDS once they put their mind to it. WE want a "cocktail" as well! In the meantime, I wish health and wellness to all on our road, and I hope this book helps you find your way!

1 ANTIBACTERIAL/ANTIVIRAL/ANTIFUNGAL

With the current ticks being so dirty today, many sufferers need a comprehensive treatment program that includes treatment for bacteria, viruses, parasites and yeast/fungus.

MULUNGU – kills bacteria

STEPHANIA – antibacterial, antiparasitic

AILANTHUS ALT. – natural antibiotic, for BARTONELLA air hunger, asthma

ARIZONA CYPRESS – antifungal, antibacterial, decreases bacterial BIOFILMS (helps destroy LYME bacteria)

SHATAVARI – natural antibiotic

BERBERINE – strengthens resistance against common illness causing bacteria, maybe C. difficile, antiparasitical

SIDA ACUTA – antimicrobial, antibacterial, BARTONELLA, MYCOPLASMA, BABESIA

BIDENS – *antibiotic*, *antibacterial*, *antimicrobial, antimalarial*, equal to the drug AMPHOTERECIN B

CHAPPARO AMARGOSA – chronic digestive inflammation, post antibiotic therapy, amoebic dysentery, giardia, intestinal protozoa, CANDIDA, bacterial enteritis, healing mucosa of the GI tract

DESERT WILLOW – for YEAST, ANTI-CANDIDA, ANTIFUNGAL

CRYPTOLEPSIS – BABESIA, anti-inflammatory (blocks Cox 2), systemic, ANTIBACTERIAL, protozoal properties, staph infections, antiparasitic, antimicrobial

ALCHORNEA – antimalarial, antibacterial, antimicrobial, antifungal, antiprotozoal, antiamoebic, anthelminthic, BABESIA, BARTONELLA, MYCOPLASMA, CANDIDA

HOUTTUYNIA – antiviral, antibacterial, antifungal, antimicrobial, anthelmintic, anti-inflammatory, Strongly active against MYCOPLASMA and BARTONELLA, removes TOXINS

MARSH WOUNDWORT - LYME flare ups

AFRICAN PEACH RT. – (Nauclea latifolia rt.) Malaria, epilepsy, broad spectrum antibiotic, specific for BABESIA, antibacterial, antiparasitic, BLOOD CLEANSER

PASQUE FLOWER – intestinal worms

MOTHERWORT – antibacterial, anti-inflammatory, MYCOPLASMA, loss of energy

ANAMU – kills bacteria, fungi, viruses, CANDIDA

EYEBRIGHT – fights harmful BACTERIA

LION'S MANE – LYME, anti-inflammatory

TEASEL – ability to pull the BACTERIA from tissues and into bloodstream, exposing it to antibiotics and immune system helps rid body of chronic LYME

GREATER CELANDINE – ANTIFUNGAL, MYCOPLASMS

JAPANESE KNOTWEED – specific for LYME and BARTONELLA, antibacterial, antiviral, antifungal, antispirochetal

CHINESE (White) PEONY – antibacterial

BLUE VERVAIN – *antimicrobial, antibacterial*

CAT'S CLAW – *antiviral* properties, fights HERPES infections, protects and repairs DNA, CANCER fighting properties

ISATIS – antimicrobial, antibacterial, antiviral (comparable to Tamiflu)

SERREPEPTASE – kills BACTERIA and promotes wound healing, kills ANTIBIOTIC RESISTANT BACTERIA, inhibits formation of BIOFILMS

ORGANIC SULFUR – CANDIDA, parasites

QUERCETIN – *antiviral,* treats common cold and influenza

2 ANTIFUNGAL/YEAST/CANDIDA

Candida/Yeast are very common infections that tag along with tick-borne diseases.

ARIZONA CYPRESS – antifungal, help dealing with respiratory molds

DESERT WILLOW – YEAST, *anticandidal, antifungal*

CHAPARRO AMARGOSA – CANDIDA, healing digestive tract

ALCHORNEA – *antifungal*

ANAMU – *antifungal*, CANDIDA

LION'S MANE – CANDIDA

TEASEL – helps treat CANDIDA overgrowth

JAPANESE KNOTWEED – *antifungal*

GREATER CELANDINE – *antifungal*, helps with MYCOPLASMS

BIDENS – *antimicrobial,* equal to the drug AMPHOTERICIN B (drug given for yeast and fungi)

ORGANIC SULFUR – CANDIDA, YEAST

3 ANXIETY/STRESS

Feeling very stressed and anxious are hallmarks of tick-borne diseases. It is hard to live any kind of life when you are so anxious. Some of the antibacterial herbs work well, but usually take time.. Not sure if it is the properties in them, or just getting the bacterial load down. I have found most of these herbs/supplements very helpful getting me through the tough times, especially until the bacterial load was down.

BOSWELLIA – may reduce anxiety and stress

SPIKENARD – *sedative,* rids mind of *anger, aggression, anxiety*

MULUNGU – anxiety (similar to VALIUM), depression, PTSD, stress, *panic disorders, insomnia, quitting Smoking*

STEPHANIA – *sedative,* specific for NERVE inflammation

SHATAVARI – anti-anxiety, may help with depression, LIBIDO/APHRODISIAC

MUIRA PUAMA – helps with stress and anxiety, helps CNS (Central Nervous System), nervous system tonic, LIBIDO/APRODISIAC, anti-fatigue

HAWTHORN – provide CALMING effect that reduces ADRENALINE

SIDA ACUTA – nervous disorders

ALBIZIA – curtails anxiety and stress, helps with depression, SUICIDAL tendencies, irrational Anger

ASTRAGALUS – helps body fight stress

HOLY BASIL (TULSI) – balances stress hormones, supports THYROID and ADRENALS

ASHWAGANDHA – reduces stress and anxiety, helps with depression, may stimulate THYROID gland

BERBERINE – anxiety

CORDYCEPS – combats stress, supports mental health

MARSH WOUNDWORT – *sedative* effect on CNS

AFRICAN PEACH RT. (Nauclea latifolia rt.) – anxiety

PASQUE FLOWER – *sedative*, anxiety, general nervous tension, PANIC ATTACKS, FEAR, DREAD, PANIC, *nervine*

JAMAICAN DOGWOOD – anxiety, *sedative*, HYSTERIA, MUSCLE SPASM

WOOD BETONY (pedicularis) – *tranquilizer, sedative,* MUSCLE RELAXANT, psychological effects, good for ANGER, FEAR, PAIN, ANXIETY

WILD LETTUCE – soothes anxiety, *sedative*

MOTHERWORT – *sedative,* reduces anxiety and sleeplessness, strong relaxant for anxiety, *heart racing* from nervous tension, strongly neuroprotective, reduces BLOOD CLOT formation

ANAMU – sedates, reduces anxiety

CORAL RT. – able to calm and relax the NERVES, especially calms HEART and MIND, HEAD, NECK, SHOULDERS, WAIST, LEGS and ARMS

LINDEN – soothes the heart, uplifts spirits, anxiety, *nervine,* tension, restlessness, PANIC ATTACKS

TEASEL – feelings of COMFORT and EXHILIRATION

LION'S MANE – anxiety, depression, cognitive function

CURCUMIN – may improve MENTAL HEALTH, BRAIN HEALTH, depression and anxiety

GYNOSTEMMA – helps control stress and anxiety level

CISSUS QUADRANGULARIS – may improve anxiety

BLUE VERVAIN – *nervine,* depression, anxiety, can promote positive thinking, stimulates increase of neurotransmitters DOPAMINE and SEROTONIN, clears mind of worry and fear

CHINESE (White) PEONY – nervousness, enhance mental function

JAPANESE KNOTWEED – CNS relaxant, CNS (brain and spinal cord) protectant, strong actions in the CNS and BRAIN, stimulates microcirculation in the BRAIN

CAT'S CLAW – anti-anxiety properties

GREATER CELANDINE – mild sedative

SCHISANDRA – helps support ADRENAL GLANDS, mood boosting, stress reducing

INOSITOL – anxiety

4 BLOOD PRESSURE/HEART/BLOOD FLOW

I, personally, have been able to use herbs and supplements successfully to deal with any heart issues that have come up.

MARAL RT. – heart health, may fight blood clots, can reduce HIGH BLOOD PRESSURE, helps with endurance, strength and recovery

MULUNGU – lowers blood pressure, heart palpitations

STEPHANIA – CALCIUM CHANNEL BLOCKER, vasodilator, antifibrotic, HYPERTENSION, cardiac disease

AILANTHUS ALT. – normalization of HEART RATE, protects VASCULAR system, blood flow and blood Pressure, regulates abnormal calcium induced rhythms in the HEART, can improve HEART FAILURE

ARIZONA CYPRESS – varicose veins, phlebitis

HAWTHORN – heart tonic, increased blood flow to the heart, strengthens contraction of HEART MUSCLE, increases circulation by dilating blood vessels which allows for increased OXYGEN delivery to tissues, reduces palpitations, provides CALMING effect that normalizes BLOOD PRESSURE, lowers LDL cholesterol, reduces adrenaline

CURCUMIN – lowers risk of heart disease, helps prevent BLOOD CLOTS

BERBERINE – optimum BLOOD PRESSURE

BIDENS – hypotensive

DESERT WILLOW – cardiovascular health

CORDYCEPS – supports heart health

KHELLA – combats spasms in the smooth muscles that line the walls of the BLOOD VESSELS, improves circulation in the HEART MUSCLE and gives mild boost for the hearts pumping action, helps prevent congestive heart failure, one of the chemical constituents (Visnagin) also acts as a CALCIUM CHANNEL BLOCKER preventing blood vessel constriction that would result in high blood pressure, two other compounds (Khellin and Visnadin) help keep blood vessels from constricting in response to EPINEPHRINE pumped from the ADRENALS during STRESS, increases ratio of HDL to LDL reducing the likelihood of cholesterol plaque formation in injured arteries

MARSH WOUNDWORT – cardioprotective

AFRICAN PEACH RT. – HIGH BLOOD PRESSURE

PASQUE FLOWER – improves blood circulation , can cure MYOCARDIUM (thickening of the cardiac Muscle), healer for HIGH BLOOD PRESSURE

JAMAICAN DOGWOOD – cardio tonic

WILD LETTUCE – hardening of the arteries

SARSAPARILLA – helps with HIGH BLOOD PRESSURE

MOTHERWORT – heart racing from nervous tension, strengthens HEART MUSCLE, *hypotensive*, slows and strengthens HEART BEAT, lowers BP, reduces BLOOD CLOT formation

CORAL RT. – stabilizes blood pressure, calms heart and mind

LINDEN – cardiovascular conditions, hyperactivity

HORNY GOAT WEED – helps with high blood pressure

SERREPEPTASE – lowers risk of ATHEROSCLEROSIS, can help stop blood clots, can help remove Calcium deposits, decrease permeability of capillaries (small blood vessels), May reduce STROKE risk, fibrinolytic properties

ORGANIC SULFUR – builds flexible cells in ARTERIES and VEINS

VINPOCETINE – STROKE prevention, almost halved the amount of plaque in the arteries, reduces Viscosity of STICKINESS of red blood cells, SODIUM CHANNEL BLOCKER

BOSWELLIA – *antithrombotic, anticoagulant* properties that regulate blood pressure, improves HDL and LDL cholesterol levels

BLUE VERVAIN – cardioprotective

CHINESE (WHITE) PEONY – normalizes blood pressure, heart benefits, THINS BLOOD

JAPANESE KNOTWEED – cardioprotective, highly protective of ENDOTHELIA, enhances BLOOD FLOW, especially to the EYES, HEART, SKIN and JOINTS, invigorating and clearing blood, reduces pulse pressure to normal

CAT'S CLAW – dilates blood vessels, normalizes blood pressure, lowers HYPERTENSION

KUDZU – Congestive Heart Failure, Heart Attacks, reduces the heart's need for OXYGEN and improves coronary circulation, relax the muscle lining in the left coronary vessel and lowers the heart rate, one compound is a BETA BLOCKER which reduces a racing pulse induced by STRESS, lowers blood pressure and helps reduce swelling in the eyes with GLAUCOMA

EVENING PRIMROSE OIL – boosts HEART HEALTH, helps prevent HYPERTENSION, anti-inflammatory, Reduces cholesterol levels

COQ10 – improves HEART health, blood pressure, CONGESTIVE HEART DISEASE, may prevent ENLARGEMENT of the HEART, may reduce HARDENING of the ARTERIES, found in high Concentrations in the HEART MUSCLE, ANGINA, HEART FAILURE

PEA – helps to prevent HEART ATTACK, helps control HYPERTENSION

QUERCETIN – high blood pressure, cardiovascular disease, METABOLIC SYNDROME

BROMELAIN – cardiovascular disease, may reduce triglycerides

ACETYL-L-CARNITINE – helps maintain cardiovascular health

B6 – may prevent clogged arteries

D-RIBOSE – supports heart health, improves myocardial energy levels

5 BLOOD SUGAR/METABOLIC SYNDROME

Even though I always had low blood sugar, blood sugar control became a problem for me after being infected by ticks. I have even read that some people develop insulin-dependent diabetes from these diseases. With the help of herbs and supplements, my fasting blood sugar is now in the normal range and I have a good A1C, which is a blood test that is 3 month marker of blood sugar control.

MARAL RT. – Metabolic Syndrome, improves blood sugar, blood fats, helps with DIABETES

CAT'S CLAW – DIABETES, insulin resistance

SHATAVARI – helps maintain blood sugar

HAWTHORN – *hypoglycemic* activity, for Type 2 diabetes

CURCUMIN – regulates blood sugar

BERBERINE – blood sugar balance

BIDENS – anti-diabetic

DESERT WILLOW – regulates glucose metabolism

CORDYCEPS – regulates blood sugar, dizziness

SIDA ACUTA – *hypoglycemic*

CRYPTOLEPSIS – *hypoglycemic*

MARSH WOUNDWORT – diabetic treatment

AFRICAN PEACH RT. – Metabolic Syndrome, antidiabetic, anti-obesity

MILK THISTLE – can result in lower fasting blood sugar levels, regulates the amount of insulin in circulation in the bloodstream

HOUTTUYNIA – regulates blood sugar, helps in weight loss, *hypoglycemic*

SARSAPARILLA – blood sugar reduction

CISSUS QUADRANGULARIS – may reduce fasting blood glucose, HBA1C, and TRIGLYCERIDES, may Improve INSULIN SENSITIVITY

EYEBRIGHT – lowers blood sugar

ANAMU – lowers blood sugar

ASTRAGALUS – treats diabetes

CHINESE (white) PEONY – may benefit diabetes and weight gain

GYMNEMA – reduces sugar cravings (makes sweet foods taste less appealing), helps lower blood sugar levels, may increase insulin levels, improves cholesterol and triglycerides levels, heart disease risk, may aid in weight loss.

HARATAKI – helps prevent diabetes, activates Beta pancreatic cells to produce INSULIN, helps breakdown of starch into glucose

ELEUTHERO – stabilizes blood sugar levels

REISHI (Mushroom) – blood sugar control

ORGANIC SULFUR – insulin production

QUERCETIN – METABOLIC SYNDROME

ACETYL – L – CARNITINE – regulates blood sugar, helps reduce symptoms of Type 2 Diabetes

6 BRAIN/DEPRESSION/NERVES

The brain can be greatly affected by all tick-borne diseases, and there have been horror stories of people being put into mental hospitals. The doctor who diagnosed me actually told me I was in a type of pre-Alzheimer state. Bartonella can be an especially cruel bacteria to the brain. Some sufferers develop PTSD from trying to find doctors that will listen to them. While treating with antibacterial drugs and herbs, these supplements have helped immensely with brain malfunctions. Some of these I will most likely will be taking for the rest of my life.

SOPHORA – may improve DEPRESSION, may treat ALZHEIMER'S, neuro inflammation

MARAL ROOT – DEPRESSION, anxiety, stress, libido, brain health, may help prevent STROKES, Improves EMOTION, may prevent INTOXICATION, improves mental health in mentally fatigued people,

SPIKENARD – relaxes body and mind, rids mind of ANGER, AGRESSION and ANXIETY, sedates feelings of depression and restlessness, NEUROPROTECTIVE, HEADACHES, DIZZINESS, VERTIGO

MULUNGU – balances NEUROTRANSMITTERS, for quitting SMOKING

EPIMEDIUM (Horny Goat weed) – *neuroprotective,* may help regenerate NERVES, may help DEPRESSION improves BRAIN BLOOD FLOW, sharpen memory, normalizes cortisol levels, boosts energy

STEPHANIA – reduces inflammation in the BRAIN, reduces CYTOKINES in the BRAIN, specific for nerve inflammation

AILANTHUS ALT. – memory loss, recalling things, concentration

SHATAVARI – may help treat depression, enhance physical stamina, for fatigued ADRENAL glands

JAPANESE KNOTWEED – strong actions in the CNS and BRAIN, specific for protecting BRAIN from NEUROTOXIC substances such as beta amyloid associated with ALZHEIMER'S, Stimulates MICROCIRCULATION in the BRAIN

HARATAKI – improves COGNITIVE functioning, improves memory capacity, FOCUS, CONCENTRATION, CALMNESS, ALERTNESS, REASONING, PROBLEM SOLVING

MUIRA PUAMA – may stop progression of ALZHEIMER'S, BRAIN TONIC, prevent cognitive impairment, decreases brain AMYLOID PLAQUE deposits, can enhance MEMORY, promotes NEURONS for memory and learning, protects NEURONS from OXIDATIVE STRESS by lack of glucose and oxygen, tonifies the nervous system, help with stress induced DEPRESSION

CURCUMIN – boost BRAIN FUNCTION, helps DEPRESSION, may improve MENTAL HEALTH, improves Memory, boosts BDNE neurotropic factor for BRAIN functions

ALBIZIA – DEPRESSION

BIDENS – neuroprotective

CORDYCEPS – slows aging and promotes clarity, improves athletic performance, supports mental health, DIZZINESS

ALCHORNEA – strong impact on BRAIN and CNS

SIDA ACUTA – DEPRESSION

SARSAPARILLA – BRAIN protection

MOTHERWORT – stops MYCOPLASMA damage in the BRAIN

ELEUTHERO – repairs nerve damage, increases blood flow to the BRAIN

EYEBRIGHT – strengthens MEMORY

CORAL ROOT – improves INTELLIGENCE, calms HEART and MIND, and relieves ANGRY feelings

LION'S MANE – DEPRESSION, memory

TEASEL – feelings of COMFORT and EXHILIRATION

CHINESE (white) PEONY – enhance MENTAL FUNCTION

BLUE VERVAIN – DEPRESSION, can promote POSITIVE THINKING, clears mind of WORRY and FEAR, stimulates release of DOPAMINE and SEROTONIN

CAT'S CLAW – may reduce amyloid deposition associated with cognitive decline

EVENING PRIMROSE OIL – helps BRAIN FUNCTION

SERREPEPTASE – helps prevent ALZHEIMER'S by reducing BRAIN INFLAMMATION

ORGANIC SULFUR – helps reverse ALZHEIMER'S, increased circulation in the BRAIN

VINPOCETINE – improves CEREBRAL BLOOD FLOW, enhances the delivery of oxygen and nutrients to the BRAIN, additional support to cope with bouts of STRESS, LOW MOODS and manage FRUSTRATION

PHOSPHATIDYLSERINE (PS) – may improve cognitive function, helps improve MEMORY, may help with ALZHEIMER'S, reduces symptoms of DEPRESSION, aids in athletic performance, may help with MOBILITY, can reduce STRESS, improves sleep quality, helps with ADHD

5-HTP – improves mood, better sleep, appetite suppressant, increases SEROTONIN so helps with DEPRESSION, works in BRAIN and CENTRAL NERVOUS SYSTEM, improves symptoms of FIBROMYALGIA, may help reduce MIGRAINE frequency. (Long term supplementation may deplete DOPAMINE, EPINEPHRINE and NOREPINEPHRINE)

CITICOLINE – boosts cognition, nootropic effects, prevents brain damage, improves EYESIGHT, may help with DEPRESSION and ADDICTION, supports STROKE recovery, increases production of NEUROTRANSMITTERS ACETYLCHOLINE, NOREPINEPHRINE and DOPAMINE, Stimulates BLOOD FLOW to BRAIN, helps improve symptoms of ALZHEIMER'S, cutting levels of Inflammation molecules (like HISTAMINE), PARKINSON'S, MS

PALMITOTLETHANOLAMIDE (PEA) – BRAIN health and regeneration, helps with symptoms of DEPRESSION

QUERCETIN – mood disorders

CoQ10 – for brain, may slow the progression of Alzheimer's and Parkinson's

ACETYL-L-CARNITINE – improves mood, learning and memory, promotes nervous system and well-being, boosts mitochondrial brain function, may reduce BRAIN and NERVE damage, combats DEPRESSION

B6 – can increase SEROTONIN and DOPAMINE

7 CIRCULATION AND LYMPHATICS

Circulation of the blood and lymphatic systems can become very congested with these diseases. Blood may become thick and lymph stagnant. These supplements have been very helpful.

CURCUMIN – helps prevent BLOOD CLOTS

MARSH WOUNDWORT – prevents deterioration of ENDOTHELIAL CELLS

PASQUE FLOWER – poor circulation

MOTHERWORT – reduce BLOOD CLOT formation

CORAL ROOT – blood circulation

TEASEL – strengthens knees and back

CHINESE (white) PEONY – THINS blood

JAPANESE KNOTWEED – *antithrombotic,* highly protective of ENOTHELIAL tissues, invigorating and clearing the blood

GREATER CELANDINE – treat blood stasis, ANTITOXIN

HORNY GOAT WEED – may improve circulation by thinning the blood

RED ROOT – Lymph

ELEUTHERO – improves LYMPHATIC FUNCTION, increases circulation

EVENING PRIMROSE OIL – helps with blood circulation

LUMBROKINASE – keeps blood flowing

SERREPEPTASE – can be used for dissolving BLOOD CLOTS, CYSTS and ARTERIAL PLAQUE, improves VEINS, breaks down SCAR tissue, may break down FIBRIN

VINPOCETINE – reduces VISCOSITY of STICKINESS of red blood cells

ACETYL-L-CARNITINE – lowers inflammation and boosts circulations

ORGANIC SULFUR – builds flexible cells in the ARTERIES and VEINS

8 CONSTIPATION

Constipation can become a huge problem with many of these diseases. It is especially problematic because you need to keep the elimination channels open in order to not have a toxin build-up that can make you sick

MAGNESIUM – constipation

VITAMIN C – to bowel tolerance for constipation

LLANTEN – constipation, appetite suppressant, curbs hunger pangs

FENUGREEK – constipation, gas

HARITAKI – constipation and other digestive issues

PSYLLIUM – fiber that regulates bowel movements

INOSITOL – constipation

9 DIGESTION

Many digestive issues can occur with the diseases and in treatment, especially when taking antibiotics and antibacterial herbs.

SHATAVARI – improves ULCERS, digestive health, HEARTBURN, indigestion, irritable bowel (IBS), diarrhea

MUIRA PUAMA – helps gastro issues, may reduce cholesterol and body fat

BERBERINE – improves digestion and microbial balance

ALBIZIA – binds water and food by speeding digestive process and keeps bowel movements regular

SIDA ACUTA – protects stomach lining

ALCHORNEA – *antidiarrheal*

MARSH WOUNDWORT – for sensitive gut (use with Bidens)

AFRICAN PEACH RT. – CONSTIPATION, reduced morning sickness, bad breath, blood cleanser, eliminates toxins

PASQUE FLOWER – digestive system

HOUTTUYNIA – GASTRITIS, DYSENTERY, *laxative*, intestinal infections

SARSAPARILLA – binds endotoxins in the alimentary canal, DETOX NICOTINE, indigestion

MOTHERWORT – protects MITOCHONDRIAL function and integrity

LLANTEN – digestion, CONSTIPATION, mouth ulcer, for overweight obese people, appetite suppression, curbs hunger pangs

TEASEL – diarrhea

CHINESE (white) PEONY – digestive system, IBS (Irritable Bowel Syndrome)

JAPANESE KNOTWEED – slightly reduces stomach acid, anti-ulcer

CAT'S CLAW – helps treat digestive problems, stomach and gut inflammation, prevent and treat ovarian cysts, repairs DNA

CISSUS QUADRANGULARIS – may protect against stomach ULCERS

MARSHMALLOW – relieves irritation of the mucous membranes, strengthens the digestive system, coats the intestinal and urinary tract linings, lowers stomach acid levels

SLIPPERY ELM – able to neutralize excess acids in the stomach and intestines, treats irritation caused by Colitis, chronic diarrhea, esophagitis, gastritis and ulcers, the mucilage soothes inflammation and stops irritation of the mucous membranes lining the stomach and intestines

FENUGREEK – used to ease digestive tract disorders, mucilages released from the herb coat the lining of the intestines and keep the stomach from emptying quickly, with the result that glucose enters the bloodstream more slowly after a meal

HARATAKI – natural blood purifier, detoxifier, aids in digestion, improving GUT health, helps break down food particles, enhances secretion of DIGESTIVE JUICES and thereby increases the absorption of essential nutrients through the intestines, constipation, GERD

GREATER CELANDINE – gastrointestinal problems

BILE SALTS – helps digest proteins and starches, helps remove toxins including heavy metals, helps absorb fat soluble vitamins A, D, E, K, protects gut from infections, may help gut infections and SIBO (antimicrobial activity in the small bowel), may enhance WEIGHT LOSS, helps with fatty stool and diarrhea, helps remove toxic substances from the body

PEA – Gut inflammation

QUERCETIN – improves triglycerides and total cholesterol, restores SOD, CATALASE and GLUTATHIONE In LIVER

BROMELAIN – protein digesting ENZYME, HEARTBURN, digestive disorders, constipation

ACETYL-L-CARNITINE – helps muscle mitochondria to burn fat and deliver energy into cells, weight loss

ORGANIC SULFUR CRYSTALS – gut's mucosal membrane is made up primarily of sulfur, promotes repair of the mucosal layer, which can help with digestive function and nutrient absorption, helps prevent Candida growth and Leaky Gut

DGL – (deglycyrrhizinated licorice) used for Leaky Gut, Ulcers, soothes and helps heal the stomach lining, indigestion, acid reflux, nausea, stomach pain, increases production of protective mucus in the stomach and esophagus, promotes and supports blood flow to digestive lining, healthy cell growth and turnover in the digest tract, Canker sores. Has an estrogen-like effect. It also lowers potassium. Do not take with fludrocortisone or any meds that lower potassium, like diuretics.

10 ENDOTHELIAL CELLS

Bartonella can negatively affect the endothelial cells. Endothelial cells line all the blood vessels, including arteries, veins and capillaries of the BRAIN, SKIN, LUNG, HEART and MUSCLES.

MARSH WOUNDWORT – prevent deterioration of ENDOTHELIAL cells

RESVERATROL JAPANESE KNOTWEED - normalizes VASCULAR ENDOTHELIA of the body, specific for LYME and BARTONELLA, enhances blood flow to the skin

COQ10 – can reverse endothelial cell damage in the blood vessels

ARGININE – helps with endothelial dysfunction especially in Bartonella. Do not take if prone to Herpes Virus

OMEGA 3 – fatty acids have beneficial effects on vascular endothelial function

POMEGRANATE – endothelial protecting mechanisms

VITAMIN E – protects endothelial function

VITAMIN C – protects from endothelial damage caused by oxidative stress

11 EXCESS IRON

I found out through DNA testing that I have a genetic issue with iron overload. Although it is only one-sided, and has a very low incidence of causing problems, because of all the tick-borne diseases, unfortunately, it did. I have come across quite a few others in different groups with this problem, so included this section. Others seem to deal with low iron/anemia. They should be very careful with these herbs and supplements.

CURCUMIN – helps to lower iron, chelates and blocks iron (curcumin cream available)

RESVERATROL – chelates and blocks iron

IP6 – blocks iron

MILK THISTLE – chelates, blocks iron

FENUGREEK – contain mucilage that interfere with iron absorption, may bind iron, as a caution it can interfere with thyroid medications

QUERCETIN – chelates, blocks iron

GREEN TEA EXTRACT – chelates, blocks

HORNY GOAT WEED – the chemical ICARIIN in Horny Goat Weed has been shown to reduce iron HARITAKI – may contain active substances capable of lessening iron overload induced toxicity, therefore useful for chelating in iron overload diseases

FIBER – helps to block iron

12 EYES

All tick-borne diseases can cause eye issues, but from everything I have read or experienced, Bartonella seems to be the infection that is the most problematic.

STEPHANIA – eye conditions with Lyme, retinopathy in diabetes, ocular involvements

AILANTHUS ALT. – blurry vision, ophthalmic disease

PASQUE FLOWER – Cataracts, Glaucoma, conjunctivitis

MOTHERWORT – decreases SENSITIVITY to LIGHT

EYEBRIGHT – helps promote HEALTHY RETINA and LENSES, eyesight, eye inflammation

LLANTEN – irritated eyes

PEA – (PALMITOYLETANOLAMIDE) supports EYE health

TEASEL – soothe sore eyes

CHINESE (white) PEONY – unclear VISION, VERTIGO

JAPANESE KNOTWEED – enhances BLOOD FLOW to the EYES, MACULAR DEGENERATION

GREATER CELENDINE – eye problems

HOUTTUYNIA – *ophthalmic*

VINPOCETINE – healthy eye function for elderly, NIGHT driving, VERTIGO, RETINOPATHY

HARATAKI – for large number of eye problems, poor vision

ORGANIC SULFUR – can alleviate EYE PROBLEMS

QUERCETIN – CATARACTS

BILE SALTS – may improve EYE HEALTH

13 FATIGUE

Overwhelming fatigue hits most of the Lyme and coinfection patients at one time or another. Killing the bacteria eventually helps with this, but in the meantime this list has proved very helpful.

CORDYCEPS – helps to strengthen people with long-term illnesses or suffer from exhaustion, boosts energy levels and endurance

CAT'S CLAW – CHRONIC FATIGUE

ELEUTHERO – fatigue, helps improve overall muscle strength and energy, may help with thyroid fatigue

ASTRAGALUS – helps improve energy levels, CHRONIC FATIGUE

SARSAPARILLA – fatigue

EPIMEBIUM (Horny Goat Weed) – may help with fatigue, may boost muscle mass

MUIRA PUAMA – anti-fatigue

REISHI (Mushroom) – fatigue and depression

RHODIOLA - fatigue

COQ10 – energy production, reduce fatigue, chronic fatigue (CFS), FIBROMYALGIA, increase muscle Power

ACETYL-L-CARNITINE – delivers energy to cells, increases endurance, prevents muscle damage, more physical and mental energy, reduces fatigue

D-RIBOSE – improves energy levels, boosts stamina, enhances exercise, helps treat FIBROMYALGIA and CHRONIC FATIGUE, decreases pain and improves sense of well being

14 GLUTAMATE/GLUTAMINE

GLUTAMATE is the main excitory neurotransmitter in the brain, GABA is the main inhibitory neurotransmitter. Some people have poor GABA conversion from Glutamine/Glutamate. Some Lyme and other tick-borne diseases have issues with this problem which can increase anxiety.

Some people have a genetic tendency for Glutamate sensitivity and imbalances of Glutamate and GABA.

MSG (monosodium glutamate) can cause headaches, muscle tightness, shortness of breath, nausea and swelling of the throat for susceptible people.

I have recently read that CAFFEINE can increase Glutamate activity and too much Glutamate can actually raise levels of HISTAMINE.

B6 – is essential in the conversion of Glutamate to GABA

SOPHORA – reduces excitotoxicity, protects CNS from GLUTAMATE, potentiates GABA

MARAL ROOT – can reduce GLUTAMATE

SARSAPARILLA – helps with overactivation of GLUTAMATE cells

VALERIAN – increases GABA by interacting with GLUTAMATE receptors to provide anxiety relief

VINPOCETINE – protective against GLUTAMATE

PQQ – blocks GLUTAMATE, makes Nerve Growth Factor (NGF), protects the brain from GLUTAMATE induced neurotoxicity

TAURINE – acts like GABA in brain, protects the brain from toxic levels of GLUTAMATE

COQ10 – exhibits potent anti-glutamate properties

VITAMIN C – helps with accidental dose of MSG consumption since it protects receptors that controlthe release of GLUTAMATE providing significant protection

L-THEANINE – modestly lowers GLUTAMATE

15 HEADACHES

Headaches were one of my worst symptoms, especially when I was on antibiotics. All tick diseases can cause differing types of headaches.

MULUNGU – headaches, muscle pain

SPIKENARD – headaches, dizziness, vertigo

AILANTHUS ALT. – congested headaches

SHATAVARI – headaches

SIDA ACUTA – headaches, sore throat, toothache, sore gums

BIDENS – headaches

CORDYCEPS – headache, dizziness

KUDZU – headaches

MARSH WOUNDWORT – headache, cramps, vertigo

AFRICAN PEACH RT. – headache

PASQUE FLOWER – headaches

CHINESE (white) PEONY – headache, migraine

EYEBRIGHT – headaches, vertigo

ORGANIC SULFUR – headaches

VINPOCETINE – headaches

CoQ10 – may reduce the frequency of headaches, migraines

16 HEAT

Heat, especially damp heat, can be a problem with certain tick-borne diseases.

AILANTHUS ALT. – ailments associated with HEAT, *dizziness, vertigo, nausea,* BARTONELLA air-hunger, clears away HEAT and DAMPNESS

SIDA ACUTA – *antipyretic*

CRYPTOLEPSIS – *antipyretic*

ISATIS – *antipyretic,* bitter, cold, cools the blood and disperses stagnation, (only use for three weeks, then take a break for a couple of weeks)

AFRICAN PEACH RT. – fever, blood cleanser

LINDEN – calms excess HEAT in the body than can lead to a sense of OVERWHELM, NERVOUS DISABILITY, and feeling UNSAFE in one's body.

JAPANESE KNOTWEED – *antipyretic* (lowers heat)

HOUTTUYNIA – *antipyretic* (lowers heat)

17 HISTAMINE/ALLERGIES/MAST CELL

Lyme and Bartonella are notorious for causing food intolerances, allergies and high histamine. These supplements have been helpful.

SOPHORA – reduces HISTAMINE, allergies, MAST CELLS

CAT'S CLAW – allergies, asthma *anti-allergenic*

BOSWELLIA – clears RESPIRATORY and SINUS infections, ASTHMA

STEPHANIA – BLOCKS HISTAMINE, anti-allergenic, bronchial asthma

BERBERINE – MAST CELL REGULATION

SIDA ACUTA – asthma, common cold, flu, HEADACHES, nasal congestion, cough, wheezing

ALBIZIA – respiratory ailments, reduces inflammation in SINUS TRACTS, helps lower MAST CELL/HISTAMINE release

BIDENS – inhibits HISTAMINE, *sore throat*, *difficulty swallowing*, *itching*, *headaches*, mucus membranes

MARSH WOUNDWORT – *antihistamine,* MAST CELL, *allergenic*

HOUTTUYNIA – *anti-histamine* support

SARSAPARILLA – allergic reactions, coughs, colds, PSORIASIS, ECZEMA

ANAMU – used to fight cold, cough, SINUSITIS, TOOTHACHE, ROOT CANAL problems

LLANTEN – colds, catarrh, SINUSITIS, bronchial allergic conditions, helps reduce mucus secretions in the airways

EYEBRIGHT – ALLERGIES, COLDS, HEADACHES, coughs, SINUSITIS, reduces catarrh and mucus discharge, Catarrh from allergic conditions affecting the EYES, middle ear, sinuses, nasal passages, HAYFEVER, upper respiratory, VERTIGO

ASTRAGALUS – prevents colds and upper respiratory infections

QUERCETIN – quells allergic reactions by preventing the multiplication of cells that secrete HISTAMINE, unlike many other allergy medications in that it acts on the cells that produce histamine rather than on the nerves that stimulate those cells

SERREPEPTASE – control HISTAMINE response, treats respiratory infections, SINUSITIS, BRONCHITIS, LYMPHATIC DRAINAGE, ear, nose, throat infections, blocked airways sinus

ORGANIC SULFUR CRYSTALS - HISTAMINE inhibitor, detoxes at cellular level, allergies to FOOD and POLLEN

PEA (Palmtoylethanolamide)- HISTAMINE release blocker, helps fight common cold and influenza

18 IMMUNE SYSTEM

Some Lyme professionals and doctors believe that building up the immune system is the most important factor in treating tic-borne infections.

CORDYCEPS- *immunomodulatory* function while enhancing overall immunity by increasing LYMPHOCYTES and NATURAL KILLER CELLS

ASTRAGALUS – protect and support the IMMUNE SYSTEM

ELEUTHERO – boosts IMMUNE SYSTEM

ANDROGRAPHIS – can modulate the innate and adaptive immune response

RHODIOLA – can increase the activity of the IMMUNE SYSTEM

TURMERIC – supports IMMUNE SYSTEM by activating many types of immune cells

CAT'S CLAW – strengthens IMMUNE SYSTEM

EPIMEDIUM (Horny Goat Weed) – boosts IMMUNE SYSTEM

CHAGA (Mushroom) – IMMUNE SYSTEM MODULATION

REISHI (Mushroom) – boosts IMMUNE SYSTEM, anti-cancer fighting abilities

LION'S MANE (Mushroom) – improves the IMMUNE SYSTEM

TRANSFER FACTORS – a group of proteins produced by the cells of the IMMUNE SYSTEM, Researched Nutritionals brand Transfer Factor Multi Immune is recommended by many Lyme Doctors

LOW DOSE NALTREXONE – IMMUNE SYSTEM modulator (compounded prescription

19 KIDNEY/BLADDER

All tick-borne diseases can affect the bladder, but Bartonella and Mycoplasma seem to have been the worst for me. Some of these herbs have helped me more than antibiotics for irritable bladder symptoms.

SOPHORA – OVERACTIVE BLADDER, improves KIDNEY function

SPIKENARD – treats bacterial infections of the BLADDER, KIDNEYS and URETHRA

MULUNGU – CYSTITIS

STEPHANIA – DIURETIC

ARIZONA CYPRESS – UTI, anti-inflammatory of the urinary tract and cleans of bacteria

SHATAVARI – helps prevent KIDNEY STONES

SIDA ACUTA – UTI, CYSTITIS, urinary disease, KIDNEY STONES

BIDENS – UTI infections

CORDYCEPS – reproductive system, BLADDER infection and urination problems

ALCHORNEA – UTI

CRYPTOLEPSIS – UTI

HOUTTUYNIA – *diuretic,* infections of the urinary passages and kidneys, genital infections, astringent, removes TOXINS with antiviral and antibiotic benefits

MARSH WOUNDWORT – KIDNEY and BLADDER sensitivity

AFRICAN PEACH ROOT – strengthens the FLOW of URINE

PASQUE FLOWER – helpful to the urinary tract

WILD LETTUCE – urinary tract problems

LLANTEN – CYSITIS, increased uric acid from KIDNEYS

TEASEL – natural DIURETIC, bladder infection, KIDNEY TONIC

BLUE VERVAIN – UTI's, KIDNEY STONES

JAPANESE KNOTWEED – DIURETIC

ORGANIC SULFUR – better KIDNEY function

VINPOCETINE – for URINARY INCONTINENCE

20 LIBIDO

Having a libido is a sign of health, and sadly, many of these tick diseases rob of us of sexual feelings of intimacy and desire.

MUIRA PUAMA – improved desire, sexual fantasies, ability to reach orgasm, in 65% of women increases LIBIDO, increases blood flow to pelvis

SHATAVARI – female reproductive health, LIBIDO, *aphrodisiac,* increases blood flow to the pelvic area, enhance physical stamina for fatigued ADRENALS

SIDA ACUTA – *aphrodisiac*

CORDYCEPS – enhances sexual function, improves athletic performance, reproductive system, low energy

WOOD BETONY – *aphrodisiac*

SARSAPARILLA – LIBIDO, hormonal balance

HARATAKI – boosts sexual health and stamina, natural aphrodisiac, helps reduce MENTAL STRESS, ANXIETY, stimulates HORMONES for LIBIDO

HORNY GOAT WEED – contains chemicals that might help increase BLOOD FLOW and improve SEXUAL function, natural VIAGRA, may increase ESTROGEN and TESTOSTERONE, normalizes CORTISOL levels

21 LIVER

The Liver has to be protected and detoxed when taking so many supplements and killing off so many bacteria. VERY IMPORTANT!

MARAL ROOT – improves biliary system, protects against intoxification

SPIKENARD – HEPATO protection

HAWTHORN – lowers LDL cholesterol

BERBERINE – lowers LDL cholesterol and triglycerides

ALBIZIA – lowers cholesterol

CORDYCEPS – lowers cholesterol

SARSAPARILLA – may protect liver, blood purifier/detox

MOTHERWORT – reduces cholesterol and triglycerides

CURCUMIN – balances cholesterol

ASTRAGALUS – protects liver

TEASEL – useful for *jaundice*

VINPOCETINE – reduces elevation of LIVER ENZYMES

REISHI (Mushroom) – may increase HDL and decrease triglycerides

CISSUS QUADRANGULARIS – may lower LAB MARKERS associated with liver injury, including ALT, AST and BILIRUBIN

CHINESE (white) PEONY – helps protect against liver and spleen damage, cholesterol lowering

MILK THISTLE – liver protection, regulates digestion of fats, stabilizes cholesterol, helps liver with Alcoholism, hepatitis

JAPANESE KNOTWEED – jaundice, hyperlipidemia

GROUND FLAXSEED – may lower cholesterol

COQ10 – reduction of LDL cholesterol, reduction of triglycerides, reduction of LpA (Lipoprotein A)

QUERCETIN – NAFLD (nonalcoholic fatty liver disease), improves triglycerides and total cholesterol, Restores SOD enzymes, CATALASE and GLUTATHIONE in the liver.

NIACIN – may lower LDL cholesterol and triglycerides, may improve high density HDL cholesterol

LACTOBACILLUS PLANTARUM – lowers LDL levels and apolipoprotein B by 28%, breaks down bile salts to decrease blood cholesterol, helps with ABDOMINAL FAT

LACTOBACILLUS REUTERI – (NCIMB 30242) has the ability to lower cholesterol levels, increases cholesterol removal from the body into the stool, and increases metabolism, breakdown of cholesterol into the liver, reduces levels of C-reactive protein (62% reduction), reduces FIBRINOGEN that causes harmful CLOTTING

22 OSTEOPOROSIS

Since most of these diseases break down collagen, Osteoporosis/bone thinning may become a very real problem.

SOPHORA – OSTEOPOROSIS, collagen induced ARTHRITIS, OAB overactive bladder

SHATAVARI – helps prevent collagen breakdown

MULUNGU – OSTEOPOROSIS

TEASEL – treats OSTEOPOROSIS and OSTEPENIA

CAT'S CLAW – helps manage degenerative BONE DISEASE

CISSUS QUADRANGULARIS – may promote growth of BONE CELLS and MINERALIZATION, may block gene expression of CYTOKINES that contribute to bone loss

EPIMEDIUM (Horny Goat Weed) – may boost bone health and muscle mass

ELEUTHERO – helps reduce OSTEOPOROSIS

EVENING PRIMROSE OIL – helps prevent OSTEOPOROSIS

ORGANIC SULFUR CRYSTALS – helps reverse OSTEOPOROSIS

SILICA – helps to make collagen for bones

HYALURONIC ACID – keeps bones well lubricated

BORON – helps with BONE STRENGTH

COLLAGEN – building skin and bone (contraindicated for most of those with HISTAMINE issues)

PROPOLIS – boosts bone health and helps heal fractures by strengthening bone density

23 PAIN

Pain is very common in tick diseases, sometimes debilitating pain. Arthritis type joint pain, muscle pain, knee pain, head pain, tooth pain, nerve pain, you name it, and it will be found among tick disease patients. Bartonella causes feet and shin pain for many as well.

BOSWELLIA - pain management, lowers inflammation and swelling, reduces joint pain and arthritis, speeds up healing from infection.

MULUNGU – pain relief, MUSCLE pain

STEPHANIA – anti-arthritic, *analgesic,* smooth muscle relaxant, specific for NERVE inflammation

AILANTHUS ALT. (Tree of Heaven) – throat pain, ear pain

SIDA ACUTA – *analgesic,* sore throat, headaches, arthritis, TOOTHACHES, SORE GUMS, TONSILLITIS

MARSH WOUNDWORT – *analgesic,* pain, BONE pain

AFRICAN PEACH RT. – pain, headache, sore throat, earache

PASQUE FLOWER – headaches, pain in genital tract, NERVE pain

JAMAICAN DOGWOOD – low BACK PAIN, MIGRAINE, NERVE pain, toothache, headache, *analgesic, narcotic,* NEURALGIA, SCIATICA, arthritis

WOOD BETONY (pedicularis) – BACK pain, joint and muscle pain, muscle cramps

WILD LETTUCE – helps relieve pain, relieves muscle and joint pain, MIGRAINES, headaches, muscle relaxant

MOTHERWORT – *analgesic*

HOUTTUYNIA - *analgesic*

EYEBRIGHT – headache, sore throat

ANAMU – reduces pain

CORAL RT. – reduces pain in GOUT

LINDEN – pain and inflammation, NEURALGIA

CURCUMIN – pain, joint pain

TEASEL – *analgesic,* for pain, anti-inflammatory especially MUSCLES, helps with LYME ARTHRITIS, strengthens knees and back

GREATER CELANDINE – pain reliever, TOOTHACHE, ULCERS

DEVIL'S CLAW – anti-inflammatory and painkilling agent, ARTHRITIS, CARPAL TUNNEL SYNDROME, has been most extensively tested and found effective for relief of LOWER BACK PAIN

KUDZU – headaches, ncreases circulation that tends to reduce MUSCLE PAIN and STIFFNESS

SERREPEPTASE – helps treat pain and inflammation, treats bone and joint infections sprains torn ligaments, carpal tunnel, improves vein inflammation, muscle inflammation, arthritis

ORGANIC SULFUR (crystals) – relieves pain, helps alleviate chronic headaches, reduces muscle Inflammation, good for HANGOVERS, helps eliminate Arthritis pain and stiffness

VINPOCETINE – headaches

BLUE VERVAIN – *analgesic,* NERVINE, arthritis, headaches, general aches and pains

CHINESE (WHITE) PEONY – *analgesic,* headache, migraine, NERVE pain

JAPANESE KNOTWEED – *analgesic*

BIDENS – headaches, arthritis

EVENING PRIMROSE OIL – eases BONE pain, minimizes BREAST pain, reduces NERVE pains (especially hands and feet), Rheumatoid arthritis

PEA – (PALMTOYLETANOLAMIDE) Pain relief, neuropathic pain, LOWER BACK pain, DENTAL pain, MIGRAINES, OSTEOARTHRITIS, FIBROMYALGIA, SCIATICA, CARPAL TUNNEL, ENDOMETRIOSIS

COQ10 – MIGRAINES

QUERCETIN – arthritis, headaches, MIGRAINES

BROMELAIN – arthritis, heartburn, tendonitis, sprained ankles, connective tissue injuries such as ACL tears, joint pain

ACETYL-L-CARNITINE – chronic pain due to nerve damage and inflammation, diabetic neuropathy, Fibromyalgia symptoms

24 SINUS/RESPIRATORY/ALLERGIES

Tick-borne diseases can exacerbate allergies, respiratory and sinus issues. Personally, although I always had allergies, I was not greatly affected until I got Bartonella.

AILANTHUS ALT – dryness of the nose, congestion of NOSTRILS, enflamed mucus membranes DIZZINESS, VERTIGO, NAUSEA

ARIZONA CYPRESS – SINUSITIS, reduced sinus inflammation, aids in the elimination of excess mucus, dealing with respiratory MOLDS, soothes PHARYNGITIS

SIDA ACUTA – NASAL Congestion, eye infections, TOOTHACHE, ITCHING

ALBIZIA – reduces inflammation in the SINUS TRACT

CORDYCEPS – bronchitis, coughs, colds, flu

CRYPTOLEPSIS – upper respiratory

HOUTTUYNIA – respiratory infections

ALCHORNEA – BARTONELLA, MYCOPLASMA, respiratory

ISATIS – treats upper respiratory infections, common cold, infections of NOSE, THROAT, SINUSES, upper respiratory tract, antiviral and can even help with SARS (COVID)

MARSH WOUNDWORT – antihistamine, allergenic

AFRICAN PEACH ROOT – soothing to throat, loss of voice, hoarseness, whooping cough, dry cough, BRONCHITIS

PASQUE FLOWER – SINUSITIS, cough, asthma, severe cough, BRONCHITIS

SARSAPARILLA – allergies, encourages healthy inflammatory response

EYEBRIGHT – SINUSITIS, allergies, sore throat, helps reduce catarrh and mucus discharge from allergic conditions affecting EYES, SINUSES and NASAL passages, HAYFEVER, upper respiratory

ANAMU – used to fight colds, cough, SINUSITIS, pain, TOOTHACHE, ROOT CANAL problems

LLANTEN – respiratory infections, colds, catarrh, SINUSITIS, bronchial allergic conditions, helps reduce mucus secretions in the airways

JAPANESE KNOTWEED – respiratory infections, expectorant

GREATER CELANDINE – cough suppressant, BRONCHITIS, pulmonary infections

CAT'S CLAW- anti-allergenic properties, relief from ASTHMA

BIDENS – inhibits HISTAMINE, itching, sore throat, mucus membrane tonic, difficulty swallowing

SERREPEPTASE – SINUSITIS, lymphatic drainage, breathe easier by breaking down mucus and making it thinner, inflammation of SINUSES and BLOCKED AIRWAYS

ORGANIC SULFUR CRYSTALS – *antihistamine*

PEA – (PALMTOYLETANOLAMIDE) HISTAMINE RELEASE BLOCKER, fights common cold

QUERCETIN – natural ANTIHISTAMINE, inhibits both influenza A and B VIRUS

BROMELAIN – allergies, SINUSITIS, BRONCHITIS

25 SKIN/ITCHING

Tick-borne diseases can wreak havoc with the skin, especially BARTONELLA. From itching, skin manifestations that resemble stretchmarks, to sores and activation of Psoriasis. Lyme and Bartonella can also destroy collagen which is vital for skin and the entire body.

ALBIZIA – healthy skin, anti-inflammatory, PSORIASIS, ACNE

BURDOCK ROOT – detoxes blood and supports CIRCULATION in the SKIN

EPIMEDIUM (Horny Goat Weed) – improves skin health

SIDA ACUTA – Itching, skin diseases

EYEBRIGHT – supports skin health, ACNE, skin irritation (external)

LLANTEN – BOILS, ACNE, BITES and STINGS, BURNS, ECZEMA, PSORIASIS

TEASEL – WARTS, sores, skin problems, applied to skin for PSORIASIS

JAPANESE KNOTWEED – repairing damaged skin, PSORIASIS, normalizes VASCULAR ENDOTHELIA, carbuncles

BIDENS – ITCHING, inhibits histamine

ISATIS – can be used for PSORIASIS and other skin conditions

HARATAKI – heals wounds and infections, antibacterial, antiviral, antifungal, internally and externally

EVENING PRIMROSE OIL – skin elasticity and firmness while maintaining hydration, reduces wrinkles, ECZEMA, PSORIASIS, ACNE, HAIR LOSS

CATUABA – may improve skin, may have anti-aging effects, may also raise SPF in sunscreen, helps Prevent SKIN CANCER

SERREPEPTASE – breaks down scar tissue

ORGANIC SULFUR CRYSTALS – aids in healthy skin, reduces WRINKLES, promotes healthy growth of HAIR and FINGERNAILS, helps increase COLLAGEN and KERATIN

COQ10 – skin health, may help skin look younger, people with lower levels of COQ10 seem to be more likely to develop SKIN CANCER

D-RIBOSE – boosts skin health, anti-aging, WRINKLES

HYALURONIC ACID – internal liquid form is useful to help with collagen loss caused by the disease, it was strongly recommended by my doctor

26 SLEEP

Restful sleep can be a big problem with many Tick-borne-diseases. "Tired and Wired" is a catchphrase many use to describe their feelings which makes for disturbed sleep. Many of these have helped me when sleeping becomes problematic. Proper sleep is so important to any kind of healing.

SOPHORA – improves sleep

SPIKENARD – relaxes BODY and MIND, *sedative,* relieves INSOMNIA

MULUNGU – HEALTHY SLEEP PATTERNS

ALBIZIA – SOUND SLEEP

CORDYCEPS – promotes RESTFUL SLEEP

PASQUE FLOWER – sleeping disorders

WOOD BETONY (pedicularis) – INSOMNIA

WILD LETTUCE – INSOMNIA, induce and maintain SLEEP

MOTHERWORT – reduces ANXIETY and SLEEPLESSNESS

VALERIAN – SLEEP issues, ANXIETY, also helps with FIBROMYALGIA because of calming effect, has even proved useful for spasmodic coughing that disturbs sleep, calming effect, may even help some with lowering high blood pressure

CORAL ROOT – improves SLEEP QUALITY

LINDEN – INSOMNIA

BLUE VERVAIN – INSOMNIA

27 PROBIOTICS FOR HISTAMINE ISSUES AND ANXIETY

<u>HISTAMINE BREAKDOWN</u>

Bifidobacterium adolescentis

Bacteroides thelaiotaomicron fragilis

Lactobacillus rhamnosus

<u>LOWER HISTAMINE</u>

B. infantis

L. gasseri

L. salivarius

L. rhamnosus (especially GG) may stabilize MAST CELLS, reduce the sensitivity of HISTAMINE and allergy associated receptors

Bifido bifidum

<u>OK FOR HISTAMINE</u>

soil-based probiotics

B. infantis

B. longum

B. breve

L. gasseri

B. bifidum

L. salivarius

L. plantarum D-1033

L. acidophilus

L. Lactis

Some probiotics can actually make HISTAMINE worse.

L. casei

L. bulgaricus

PROBIOTICS FOR ANXIETY AND DEPRESSION

B. longum (may reduce depression and anxiety, helps with IBS)

B. bifidum (helps generate vitamins such as K and B12, which may also influence mood)

B. infantis (may help relaxation and treating IBS)

L. reuteri (anti-pain effect and help increase excitability?!)

L. plantarum (significantly increased SEROTONIN and DOPAMINE and reduces anxious behavior)

L. helveticus (decline in anxiety scores)

L. acidophilus (help reduce cholesterol and support nutrient absorption)

28 MISCELLANEOUS

BARTONELLA with chronic inflammation affects DOPAMINE levels to reduce motivation

UVA URSI, BERBERINE, GOLDENSEAL, BIDENS and MARSHMALLOW are useful for urinary tract infections and bladder irritations. BARTONELLA can cause a lot of bladder discomfort.

HARITAKI (Terminalia chebula) while an excellent herb for many different things, is hot in nature and too much may cause dehydration. I found that out for myself when all of a sudden my lips got dry and I started urinating more. I stopped for a couple of weeks and went back at a lower dose.

B-vitamins are important for most infections

PROPOLIS Another name for Propolis is "bee glue" and it is very helpful for managing tick-borne diseases, especially Bartonella. It purportedly helps to eliminate biofilms with yeasts, fungi, Lyme. It is antibacterial, antimicrobial, antifungal, antiviral, antiprotozoal, anti-inflammatory, antioxidant, antiseptic, antihepatotoxic and anticancer. Propolis kills bacterial and viruses by stopping their growth and spread. Fights yeast infections by blocking the growth of yeast and fungus. Helps with allergies by blocking the release of histamine. Lowers blood pressure by lowering the activity of tyrosine hydroxylase, an enzyme that can cause high blood pressure. Propolis helps the body deal with EMF radiation from electronic equipment like cell phones. It can lower blood sugar levels and protects the liver from toxins. Can be useful for tooth and oral health. It has been reported to neutralize cavities by killing bacteria and useful for gum health. Many of us have had dental horror stories from tick-borne diseases.

IODINE Tick-borne diseases can affect many with thyroid issues, IODINE is needed for the thyroid health and many other health issues. Iodine is present in breast tissues and may help prevent breast cancer, and can reduce breast pain. Helps to detox halogens such as Bromide, Fluoride, Chlorine and Bromine. Increases IMMUNE

FUNCTION, good for NERVOUS SYSTEM and BRAIN HEALTH, improves cognitive abilities, improves HAIR GROWTH, healthy HAIR, SKIN and TEETH and dry flaky skin, increases energy levels, protects from RADIATION, protects from PATHOGENS, supports REPRODUCTIVE ORGANS, helps detoxify HEAVY METALS, helps stabilize BLOOD SUGAR, some say putting iodine on a tick or mosquito bite to prevent diseases. I have taken it for years on the advice of my Lyme doctor. Definitely check with your doctor first.

LYSINE for LYME disease, helps prevent osteoporosis, helps reduce BLOOD PRESSURE, may be beneficial in reducing BLOOD SUGAR, PAIN management, reduces STRESS and ANXIETY, may help reduce CORTISOL, may help with muscle loss, FATIGUE, promotes wound healing, carries Carnitine for growth and long chain fatty acids for MITOCHONDRIA, increases calcium absorption, supports healthy gut, including LEAKY GUT, encourages COLLAGEN production, might help kill CANCEROUS growths, TMJ, BALANCE issues, NEUROPATHY, CANKER and COLD SORES (HERPES infections), MIGRAINES, EYE FLOATERS, ringing in the ears, may help RA, LUPUS and MS, ECZEMA, NODULES and CYSTS, THYROID problems, inhibits and deters SHINGLES, EPSTEIN BARR and other pathogens, by inhibiting and reducing pathogen load, L-Lysine acts as an anti-inflammatory to the entire nervous system and the VAGUS and PHRENIC nerves which are targeted by neurotoxins produced by EBV, SHINGLES and other bugs, Can be taken with ARGININE to normalize hormonal response in HIGH TRAIT ANXIETY, strengthening BONES and increasing GROWTH HORMONE

ARGININE is useful for BARTOMELLA. According to the herbalist Stephen Buhner, ARGININE has been found to reverse many of the effects of a Bartonella infection because it is specifically protective of ENDOTHELIAL cells from the kind of damage the bacteria causes. Reduces CYTOKINE cascade the bacteria initiates and stops from preventing more. Can lower blood sugar levels and blood pressure. May help to control cortisol levels. DO NOT take if you have shingles or any type of herpes. In some people it may worsen allergies and asthma.

DIET is very important for most people with tick-borne diseases, especially since many of them develop allergies or intolerances. Myself, and many I know, are gluten, dairy and sugar free.

LYME

Japanese Knotweed

Cat's Claw

Sida Acuta

Bidens

Cryptolepsis

Alchornea

Isatis

Kudzu

Stephania

Ailanthus altissima

Chinese Skullcap

Chinese Senega

Greater Celandine

Anamu

Propolis

A-L Complex Byron White

BLT, Researched Nutritionals

Cowden Protocol (Banderol, Cumanda, Samento, Stevia, Quina, Tangarana)

Jernigan Protocol

MYCOPLASMA

Cordyceps

Chinese Skullcap

Isatis

Houttuynia

Sida Acuta

Schisandra

NAC (N-Acetylcysteine)

Vitamin E

Olive Oil (1 oz AM and 1 oz bedtime)

Multi-vitamin

Myco P Researched Nutritionals

BARTONELLA

Japanese Knotweed

Houttuynia

Sida Acuta

Cat's Claw

Cordyceps

Red Root

Hawthorn

Milk Thistle

Black Walnut

Cryptolepsis

Propolis

EGCG

Quercetin

L-Arginine

A-Bart, Byron White

MC-BAR 1 and 2, Beyond Balance

BLT, Researched Nutritionals

Cowden Protocol (Banderol, Houttuynia, Samento, Tangarana)

David Jernigan Protocol

<u>BABESIA</u>

Cryptolepsis

Chinese Skullcap

Bidens

Artemisinin

Red Sage

Sida Acuta

A-Bab, Byron White

Cowden protocol (Banderol, Enula, Houttuynia, Quina, Tangarana, Chanca Piedra)

<u>DETOXIFICATION</u>

Bentonite Clay (adding psyllium fiber helps)

Activated Charcoal

Organic Sulfur

Glutathione

Zeolite

Fiber

Infra-red sauna

<u>BIOFILMS</u>

Lumbrokinase

Serrepeptase

Avea (Cowden)

Stevia

Cistus Tea

Many of these herbs and supplements can be found on Amazon. Others not on Amazon can be bought on-line through Sage Apothecary and Wise Woman Herbals. More obscure ones can be found on Etsy. Etsy does a great job and some offer free shipping.

Elk Mountain Herbs has been the only place I have been able to find Pasque Flower (Pulsatilla patens). I have only found the herb Sophora (Sophora flavescens), also known as Ku Shen, from Secrets of the Tribe.

Some Lyme doctors, like Dr. Marty Ross, sell many herbs and supplements on their websites. His website sells all the Researched Nutritionals products and other cutting-edge products and information. He also offers free shipping on orders over a certain amount.

Forrest Health website offers the Byron White formulas.

More companies are now offering the option of glycerin tinctures instead of alcohol. Some people have problems with tolerating alcohol. I have heard a rumor that the glycerin tinctures are not as effective as alcohol, but I have been ordering more of them when I find them. I am not totally sure if that is true, and unless I find out for sure I will be using them. Alcohol, though, can be diminished to a large degree by heating (but not boiling) the water before adding the tincture, and letting them sit for a while. It helps to evaporate the alcohol.

Sage Apothecary also carries some of their herbs in pill form.

Some herbal companies are offering tinctures and pills with multiple herbs, so you don't have to buy so many different products. Those come in very handy when you are dealing with antibiotic herbals and herbs for the nervous system. But it is harder to root out a single herb that could be causing a reaction. I've had a couple I can't take, like Andrographis. It made me itch and gave me a rash. Only a very small percent get that type of reaction. But now I know I won't buy any herbal combination that has Andrographis on the label. All in all, I have done very well with herbs, but very occasionally will get a reaction. I can only think of a few.

There is a company called Samsara Herbs that has a couple of multi-herbal products that many have successfully used. One is called Tick Immune Support. They changed the product and now it contains Andrographis, so I no longer purchase it. But, like I said, I am the exception with Andrographis. They have another product called Samsara Herbs Biofilm Formula, which is a very useful product.

INDEX

Q

R

S

T

V

W

Z

Made in the USA
Monee, IL
18 March 2025

14232861R00042